HOW TO LOSE WEIGHT FAST WITHOUT EXERCISING

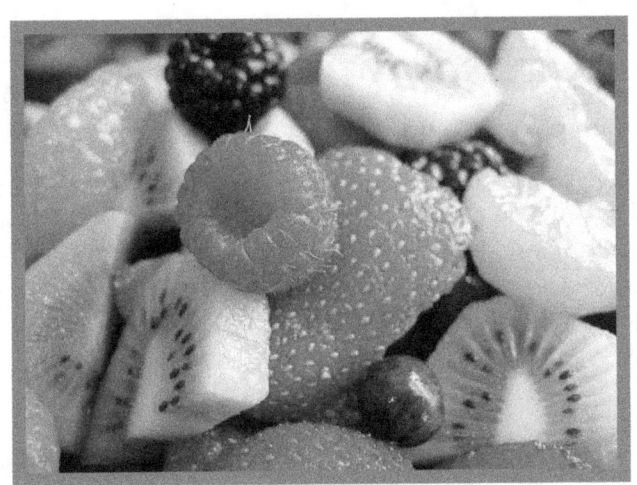

Written By:

Dr. Kathleen B. Oden
Certified Health Minister
Certified Essential Oil Coach

Create Anewu Health Ministry

Create Anewu Health Ministry©

HOW TO LOSE WEIGHT FAST WITHOUT EXERCISING

PART 1 - MAKE A PLAN

The fastest way, to lose weight fast is to eat every 2-3 hours. The first time I heard that, I thought they were crazy. But since I love to eat, that was no problem for me.

And, after I tried it, I realized ok, this is working. I was losing about 2-3 pounds a week or 10-12 pounds a month. And in 3 months, I had lost 40 pounds.

I ate from 8am to 8pm, however, I did eat breakfast and lunch, because I was still working at the time, not retired. But by the time I went home at 4pm, I was so full, I did not want to see any food.

But I continued to eat, because it is very important to eat every 2 hours.

SEE SAMPLE PLANS

8AM   -   bottle of water

10AM   -   bottle of water

12PM   -   large salad

2PM   -   bottle of water

4PM   -   1/2 cup soup with 3
                crackers

6PM   -   large green smoothie
                (16oz.)

8PM   -   veggie or fruit snack
(carrot sticks, apples...etc)

SAMPLE PLAN-B

8AM - breakfast & bottle of water

10AM - snack

12PM - lunch & bottle of water

2PM - bottle of water

4PM - snack
(carrot sticks, apples...etc)

6PM - fruit smoothie (16oz.)

8PM - 1/2 cup soup with 3 crackers

I learned that our body automatically looks for food every 2-3 hours. We have to "trick" the body so that it will not go into "I'm hungry mode" by sending a signal to your brain that tells you to go eat.

Eating every 2-3 hours will put a stop to the "I'm hungry mode" and it will cause your body to go into the "fat burning mode."

When we eat every 2-3 hours, our body says, "ok cells, unlock the fat and let it go and hurry up and get rid of all this food that keeps coming in here." Our body starts working overtime and even triple time, to get rid of fat, as fast as it can.

This is what causes your metabolism to speed up. And therefore, you lose weight automatically. I can only recommend or make suggestions on what and/or how much you are to eat. You will have to make your own plan, using the plans in this book, as an example.

You should try to eat all big meals before 3pm. However, I recommend snacking instead of eating large meals. After 3pm eat soup, smoothies and snacks. And also, try not to drink anything after 3pm. Try to keep your total calorie intake to 1200-1500 calories, a day and take your vitamins.

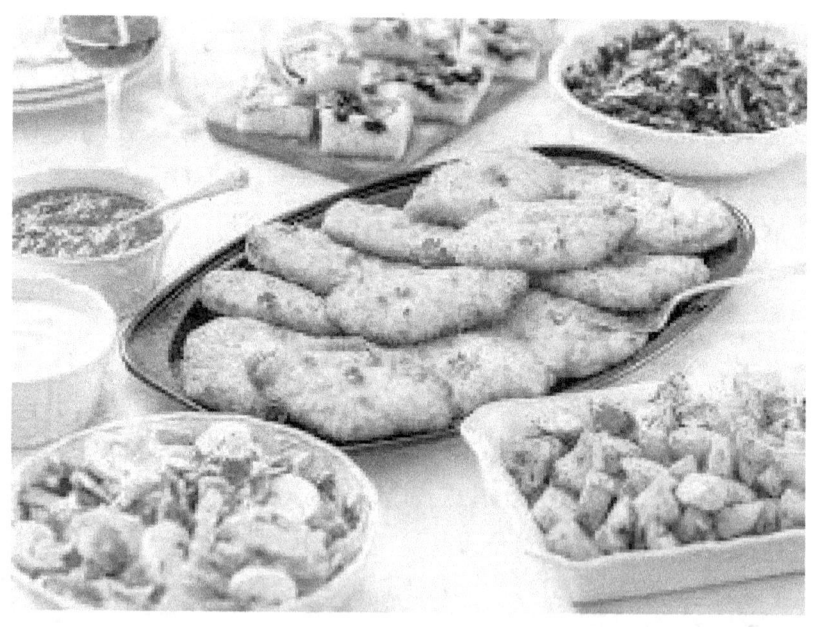

CREATING A MONTHLY PLAN

Review the following monthly plans and then create your own. You must try to evolve every 1-2 months to the next level. The following plans show you how to replace and/or eliminate, things from your diet.

Just like exercising, you cannot keep doing the same thing, over and over. You must go to the next level in order to keep losing weight.

The following plans will show you how to create your own plans so that you can continue to move forward with your weight loss plan.

Don't procrastinate, make a plan. It is better to make a plan so that you can be prepared and plan ahead. When you plan ahead, it becomes easier and easier, for you to stay on track with your new healthy eating lifestyle.

Don't procrastinate, make a plan!

<u>MONTH 1</u>

CREATE A FOOD LIST OF THINGS YOU LIKE
START PREPARING YOUR KITCHEN
START JUICING 2 DAYS A WEEK
START EATING MORE VEGGIES & FRUITS
ELIMINATE 1 THING
REPLACE 1 THING
DECIDE WHAT YOU WILL ELIMINATE IN MONTH 2
DECIDE WHAT YOU WILL REPLACE IN MONTH 2

EAT EVERY 2 HOURS
EAT FROM 8AM TO 8PM

EAT LARGE MEALS BEFORE 3PM @ (10AM, 12PM OR 2PM)

SNACKS ONLY @ (4PM, 6PM & 8PM)

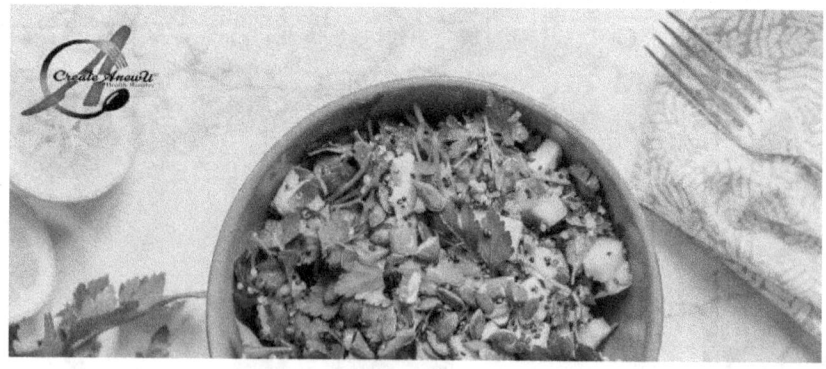

<u>MONTH 2</u>

JUICE 3 DAYS A WEEK
START EATING MORE VEGGIES & FRUITS
ELIMINATE 1 THING
REPLACE 1 THING
DECIDE WHAT YOU WILL ELIMINATE IN MONTH 3
DECIDE WHAT YOU WILL REPLACE IN MONTH 3

EAT EVERY 2 HOURS
EAT FROM 8AM TO 8PM

EAT LARGE MEALS BEFORE 3PM @
(10AM, 12PM OR 2PM)

SNACKS ONLY @ (4PM, 6PM & 8PM)

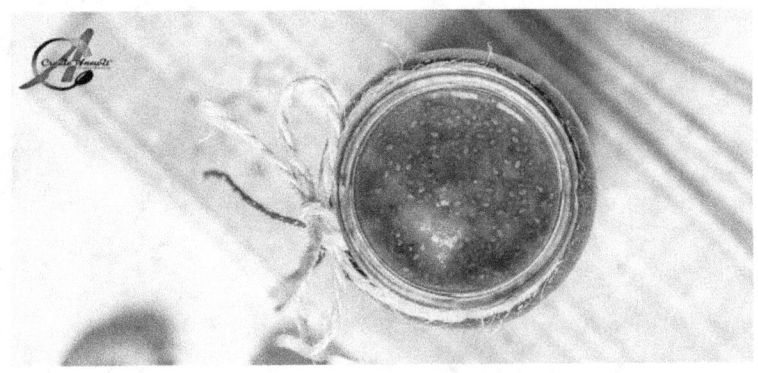

<u>MONTH 3</u>

JUICE 4 DAYS A WEEK
START EATING MORE VEGGIES & FRUITS
ELIMINATE 1 THING
REPLACE 1 THING
DECIDE WHAT YOU WILL ELIMINATE IN MONTH 4
DECIDE WHAT YOU WILL REPLACE IN MONTH 4

**EAT EVERY 2 HOURS
EAT FROM 8AM TO 8PM**

**EAT LARGE MEALS BEFORE 3PM @
(10AM, 12PM OR 2PM)**

SNACKS ONLY @ (4PM, 6PM & 8PM)

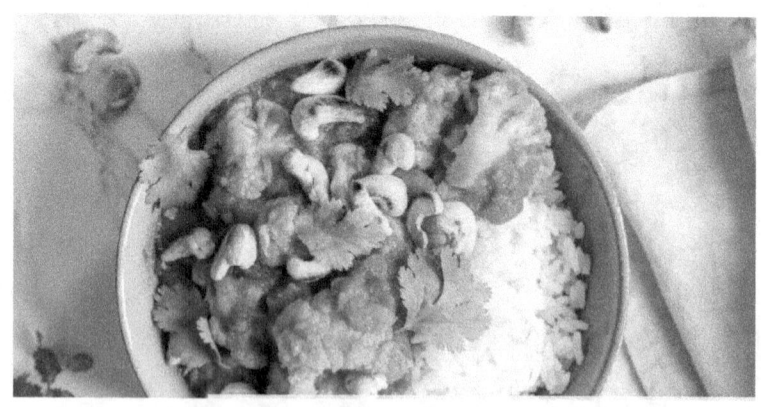

Create Anewu Health Ministry©   9

HOW TO LOSE WEIGHT FAST WITHOUT EXERCISING

PART 2 - JUCING & SMOOTHIES

Another way to lose weight fast is to juice. And it is one of the best and fastest ways to create new cells.

Try to start every morning with 2 smoothies. 8 ounces of water will make a 16 ounce smoothie. Veggies have a lot of water in them.

Create a green smoothie and a carrot smoothie. This is a powerful duo. This will kick start your day with power.

These veggie smoothies will go directly to your cells and start creating new stronger cells immediately.

Mix spinach, kale and collard greens to make a "energy power smoothie."

Add 1 collard leaf, 1 mustered or turnip leaf, 3 spinach and 2 kale to 8-16 ounces of water. Do the same with some carrots. Add 1-2 carrots to 8-16 ounces of water.

This is also a good afternoon pick-me-up and/or if you have a busy evening planned, this dynamic powerful duo is for you!

Back up your juicing with a powerful salad also made of greens. Chop up the greens and make a salad by adding your favorite veggies like tomatoes, cucumbers, or whatever you like on your salad.

This will not only keep the power going, but it will also keep you going and going and going!

No one should wake up hungry. If we are eating right our body should be full of the vitamins and minerals we need.

Drinking lots of water will also help you to lose weight fast.

TRY THESE SMOOTHIE RECIPES

Here is a HYDRATION SMOOTHIE:

CUCUMBER
CELERY
LEMON
APPLE
KALE

KILL YOUR CRAVINGS SMOOTHIE:

SWEET POTATO
LEMON
PEAR

WEIGHT LOSS SMOOTHIE:

LEMON
APPLE
KALE
CUCUMBER

HOW TO LOSE WEIGHT FAST WITHOUT EXERCISING

PART 3 - RAW POWER

When a car has the right fuel and oils, it runs better, and smoother and lasts longer.

When our body has the right food, vitamins and minerals and nutrients, we feel better, have more energy and live longer.

Juicing is number 1 and eating **RAW** is number 2, when it comes to getting the most nutrition from your fruit and veggies . Eating **RAW** veggies is always better than cooked.

Our body is made of millions and millions of cells. And the condition of the cells determines the condition of our body. If the cells are weak or damaged, due to no or low levels of vitamins and nutrients, then we are weak and sickly. And we feel tired and run down.

But, we can create new stronger cells by eating **RAW** foods that are packed with vitamins, minerals, nutrients and live enzymes.

The most powerful foods are the **RAW** green leafy vegetables, like collard green, mustered greens, turnip greens, spinach and kale.

Eating **RAW GREEN** veggies helps us to regain our strength and energy, repair our immune system and get rid of inflammation!

This can happen in 1-2 weeks or months. It all depends on the current status of your health and how much of these powerful green leafy vegetables you add to your diet.

Your main goal is to lower the chemicals in your body (eat these foods less) and raise the vitamins and minerals in your body by eating more **RAW fruit and veggies**.

Some veggies like broccoli, carrots and sweet potatoes, can be steamed. In fact, there are certain nutrients in these veggies that can only be release by steaming.

Add some baked or steamed fish and brown rice to some steamed veggies and WOW! A YUMMY HEALTHY MEAL!

Steamed sweet potato with honey and cinnamon...mmmmm good!

Purchasing an insulated lunch bag, box or tote is a good investment. Especially if you are a busy person on the go.

Take your fruits and veggies with you!

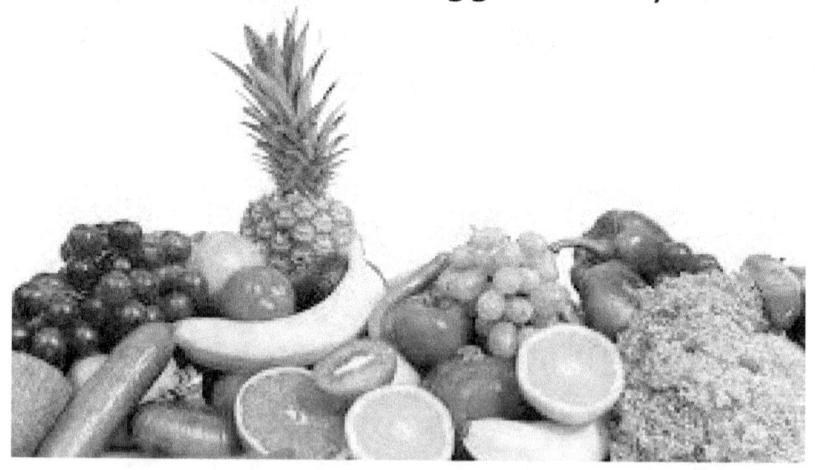

HOW TO LOSE WEIGHT FAST WITHOUT EXERCISING

PART 4 - PREPING

Mix and match, not only your daily meals but also your weekly meals. This is why you need to create a plan.

If you continue to eat the same things all the time, it will become boring and you will be tempted to go back to your old eating habits.

Stay focused and create a plan every week or for the month (which is better). This will also help you to plan ahead and create a shopping list.

Being prepared is a vital part of losing weight. Use your plan and your shopping list to plan and coordinate your meals.

Remember, it is imperative to mix and match! DO NOT create the same eating plan over and over.

Another way to be prepare is to pre-chop the items you use on a daily basis, like onions, garlic, tomatoes, cucumbers etc...

Also, cooking extra food and freezing it is a huge time saver on days you are busy.

Frozen bananas make wonderful smoothies. And buying extra avocados to freeze is very helpful. Be sure to peel bananas and avocados before freezing.

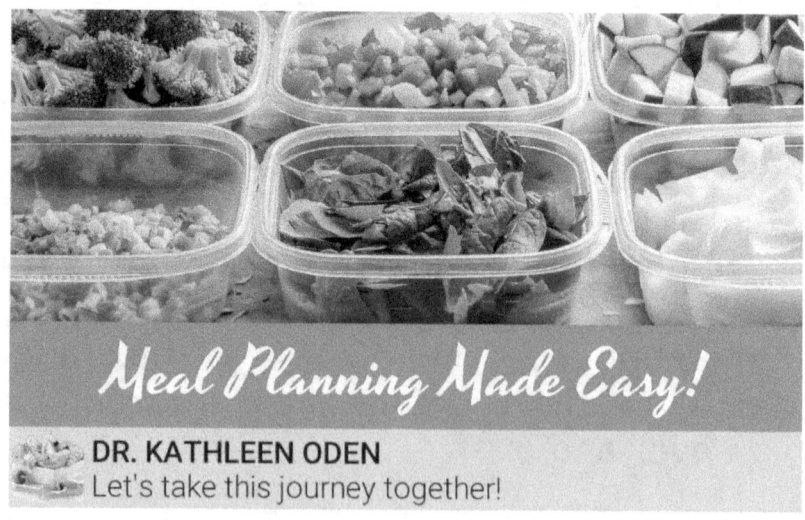

Meal Planning Made Easy!

DR. KATHLEEN ODEN
Let's take this journey together!

HOW TO LOSE WEIGHT FAST WITHOUT EXERCISING

REMEMBER THESE 3 IMPORTANT TIPS

1. Plan ahead!

2. Eat large meals before 3pm. (snacking is better)

3. Always keep to-go foods on hand. Like rasins, apples, bananas, grapes, berries, watermelon...etc.

MAKE IT HEALTHY

You can make your favorite meals healthier by adding a few RAW living foods that can add flavor and nutrition.

REAL food has enzymes. We need enzymes to help digest dead cooked food to prevent indigestion, and/or acid reflux or develop stomach problems.

REMEMER...

1. MAKE A PLAN
2. HAVE A SMOOTHIE 3-4 TIMES A WEEK
3. EAT RAW FOOD 4-5 TIMES A WEEK
4. PREP, PREP AND PREP

3 JOHN 1:2

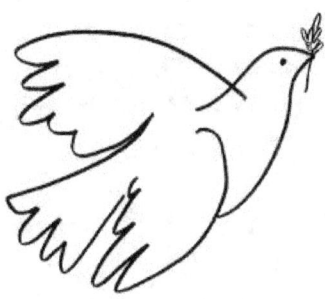

Beloved, I wish above all things that
thou mayest prosper
and be in health,
even as thy soul prospereth.

Dr. Kathleen B. Oden

Dr. Kathleen B. Oden is an author, missionary and Bible teacher, at God's House of Refuge Church & School of Evangelism. She attained a Doctorate degree in Christian Theology in 2000. Dr. Oden is a Certified Health Minister and a Certified Essential Oil Coach.

In 2015 God gave her a ministry called, Create AnewU Health Ministry. She loves ministering to people and her health ministry has opened the door for her to share what the WORD OF GOD has to say, about eating healthy food.

She has published over 20 books through Amazon.com and several of them are about health and wellness.

Dr. Oden is currently working on a book called The Old Testament Synopsis, which will be published in 2023.

1998
THE HOLY SPIRIT (Masters Degree Thesis)
2000
About The Bible (Doctorate Degree Thesis)
2004
The Old Testament (Synopsis)
2005
What God Commanded - published:2015
2006
The New Testament (Synopsis)
2012
>Hebrew Training Manual & Workbook - published:2015
>Aleph-Bet Story & Workbook - published:2015
>Biblical Hebrew & Aleph-Bet Workbook - published:2015
2015
>All About The Bible - published:2015
>21 Day Weight Loss Challenge (3 book series) - published:2015
>Create A New You In Only 90-Days - published:2015
>How To Lose Weight Fast Without Exercising - published:2015
2016
>Healthy Eating, Weight Loss & Wellness - published:2016
>3 Day Energizing & Cleansing Detox - published:2016
>How To Use Essential Oils - published:2016

REVELATION 22:2

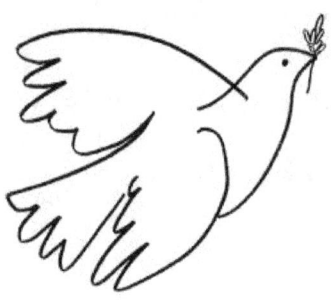

*In the midst of the street of it,
and on either side of the river,
was there the tree of life,
which bare twelve manner of fruits,
and yielded her fruit every month:
and the leaves of the tree were for the
healing of the nations*